Table of Contents

What is Keto diet?

Keto diet is a way to get your body in shape, crop the muffin top and fortify your immune system by eating plenty of fats and protein. All you have to do is drop carbohydrates, but that's much harder than it sounds. Carbohydrates (carbs) are the most abundant energy source in nature for animals across species. For example, cellulose found in plants is a carb, which is how herbivores get their calories. Insects have carbs in their carapace too, called chitin.

The problem isn't that carbs exist, it's that the way we're using them causes a lot of long-term health problems. Carbs in nature come bundled with vitamins and minerals, but processed foods we eat have refined carbs that overload the body, exhaust the pancreas and literally cause addiction. The goal of a Keto diet is to get your carb intake to 20 grams or less a day while switching you over to wholesome, healthful carbs.

What is Keto-adaptation?

Keto-adaptation is a slow and arduous process of weaning your body off of carbs and getting onto protein and fats as fuel sources. The human body is a wonderful machine that can use carbs, protein, and fats as energy with equal ease. The problem is that the body adapts to the diet we eat as kids and comes to enjoy and crave it whether it's healthy or not. So, if you've been eating cereal and drinking fizzy soda throughout your childhood, there's a good chance you'll become a lifelong consumer of those same products and brands simply because they bring you back to that time of innocence and enthusiasm.

An abundance of refined carbs also tends to turn your body into breeding grounds for all sorts of bacteria, leading to persistent infections. Keto-adaptation involves changing how you think, feel and act about and around food at the very core of your being. Rather than looking at processed carbs and their overwhelming sweetness as something that soothes and calms down, you will understand exactly what they do to your brain, mind, and heart, changing yourself from inside out and outside in.

What should I eat?

There is no officially sanctioned list of foods you must eat. Keto vegetarian diet actually puts you in charge of your menu and asks you to take responsibility for sticking to it.

All keto vegetarian dietary advice you come across is simply a suggestion to get you on the right track, but you are meant to inform yourself about the foods around you and make rational choices, sometimes on the spot. Don't fret if you falter, just keep going.

The main idea is to eat as many wholesome and unprocessed vegetarian foods as possible. Even if they aren't strictly keto, these natural foods will help your taste buds settle down and get used to what the real food is like. After that, you will find yourself adding powerful spices, such as ginger and garlic, without any prompting. Then start slowly cutting out carbs, bit by bit, until you come to the point where you don't even mind not having any throughout the day.

What is the difference between a low-carbohydrate diet and a ketogenic diet?

A keto diet is a tall order for someone who has been overloading on carbs their entire life. For such people, a low-carb diet is probably the best way to start. With it, the goal is to simply keep the carb intake steady and lower it over the course of months. There is no need to rush anything or set deadlines since carb withdrawal is a real thing and often leads the person to reach for sweets and sink into carb stupor all over again.

Both low-carb and keto diet achieve the same thing, only at different speeds. If we had to attach a number to each, we could say a low-carb diet allows for up to 50 grams of carbs a day, while a strict keto diet only allows 20 grams a day. Again, don't worry if these two numbers seem impossible to achieve, simply take your time and whittle down the carb count until you get there.

Do I need to count calories? Do calories matter?

Calories do matter, but not to the point where you have to track down every single one. You should know approximately how many calories your food contains and where they come from (carbs, protein, fats) but more than that will probably just trouble and burden you. However, pay close attention to the product labels on store-bought food and make sure you know what you're eating at all times. In other words, if the information is readily available, count everything; if not, a guesstimate will do.

How long does it take to get to ketosis?

You will feel the first effects of ketosis after a couple days, but to make a thorough change on cellular level will take months or even years. There is no way to rush this process, so relax and enjoy the adventure of discovering a whole new universe of flavors and aromas.

How often and how much should I eat?

You should eat whenever you're hungry and break up meals into smaller portions whenever possible. An exception to this is when you know you'll physically exert yourself, such as before jogging or lifting weights. Ideally, that's when you want to have a meal plan and eat a decent meal so your muscles don't waste away. The rest of the time you want to eat as little as possible, so experiment with different bite-sized portions and see how long they suppress your hunger.

How much weight could I lose and how fast?

Weight loss is tricky business since 40-50% of body weight is water, so dieters often confuse dehydration with actual loss of body fat. When you stop eating carbs you'll experience a quite sudden drop in weight of about 7 kilograms (15 pounds) during 1-2 months, since carbs tend to bind water to themselves during and after digestion. If you go back to your previous carb intake, the weight will come right back with a bit extra, so don't celebrate just yet. You ideally want to keep track of your waist circumference and work towards shaping your body through proper diet and exercise over the course of years and decades.

In next chapter, we prepared for you 60 Keto 5 Ingredients Cookbook. We hope you'll enjoy in this healthy diet.

APPETIZERS

Braised Brussels Sprout Appetizer (Crock Pot)

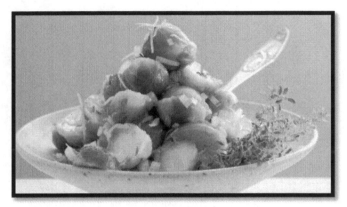

Ingredients

- 1/4 cup butter grass-fed
- 1 1/2 lbs Brussels sprouts
- 2 cloves garlic, sliced
- 2 Tbsp fresh thyme, chopped
- Salt and ground black pepper to taste
- 1/2 cup water

Instructions

1. Wash and clean the Brussels Sprout in cold water to remove any dust or dirt. Trim the top of the stem and discard it.
2. Pour the olive oil in your Crock Pot.

3. Place Brussels Sprout in your Crock Pot along with remaining ingredients; stir well.
4. Cover and cook on HIGH for 1 - 2 hours or on LOW for 3 to 4 hours.
5. Before serving drop some more butter and serve.

Servings: 6

Cooking Times

Total Time: 4 hours

Nutrition Facts

Serving size: 1/6 of a recipe (6 ounces)

Percent daily values based on the Reference Daily Intake (RDI) for a 2000 calorie diet.

Nutrition information calculated from recipe ingredients.

Amount Per Serving

Calories 118,88

Calories From Fat (59%) 70,47

% Daily Value

Total Fat 8,03g 12%

Saturated Fat 4,93g 25%

Cholesterol 20,34mg 7%

Total Carbohydrates 10,68g 4%

Fiber 4,44g 18%

Sugar 2,51g

Protein 4,02g 8%

Cheesy Swiss chard Dip (Crock Pot)

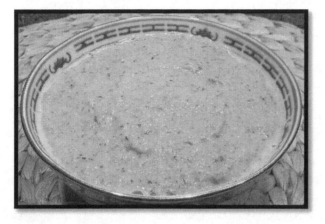

Ingredients

- 2 cups Swiss chard leaves (frozen or raw)
- 1 green onion finely chopped
- 2 cloves garlic (finely minced)
- 2 cups Cheddar cheese, grated
- 1/2 cup coconut milk (canned)

Instructions

1. Oil the bottom of your Crock Pot and lay Chard, green onion, garlic and stir well. Sprinkle grated Cheddar cheese on the top.
2. Cover and cook on HIGH 3-4 hours or on LOW for 6-8 hours.
3. Transfer Swiss chard mixture to your blender, and add the coconut milk. Blend until creamy and soft.

4. Serve hot or cold.

Servings: 4
Cooking Times
Total Time: 6 hours
Nutrition Facts
Serving size: 1/4 of a recipe (4 ounces)
Percent daily values based on the Reference Daily Intake (RDI) for a 2000 calorie diet.
Nutrition information calculated from recipe ingredients.
Amount Per Serving
Calories 300,71
Calories From Fat (73%) 218,1
% Daily Value
Total Fat 24,94g 38%
Saturated Fat 16,6g 83%
Cholesterol 69,3mg 23%
Sodium 450,92mg 19%
Potassium 180,77mg 5%
Total Carbohydrates 2,7g <1%
Fiber 0,42g 2%
Sugar 0,65g
Protein 17,21g 34%

Flourless Kale and Mozzarella Frittata (Crock Pot)

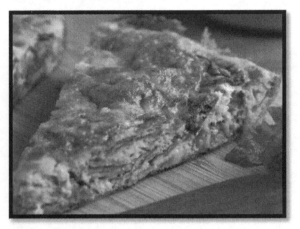

Ingredients

- 2 cup kale
- 2 green onion, sliced
- 8 eggs preferably organic
- 1/2 cup Mozzarella cheese
- 2 Tbsp olive oil
- Salt and fresh-ground black pepper to taste

Instructions

1. Pour the oil into your Crock Pot and lay chopped Kale, green onions with the pinch of salt.
2. Whisk the eggs with salt and pepper in a bowl, and pour over other Kale; stir.
3. Sprinkle crumbled Mozzarella cheese on the top.

4. Cover and cook on LOW for 2 - 3 hours.

5. Let cool for 10 minutes, slice and serve.

Servings: 6

Cooking Times

Total Time: 3 hours and 5 minutes

Nutrition Facts

Serving size: 1/6 of a recipe (3,8 ounces).

Percent daily values based on the Reference Daily Intake (RDI) for a 2000 calorie diet.

Nutrition information calculated from recipe ingredients.

Amount Per Serving

Calories 154,43

Calories From Fat (62%) 95,19

% Daily Value

Total Fat 10,67g 16%

Saturated Fat 4,18g 21%

Cholesterol 259,13mg 86%

Sodium 244,63mg 10%

Potassium 213,97mg 6%

Total Carbohydrates 3,61g 1%

Fiber 0,58g 2%

Sugar 0,88g

Protein 10,98g 22%

Mustard Cauliflower Appetizer (Crock Pot)

Ingredients

- 1 cup almond flour
- 1 tsp garlic minced
- 1 large head of cauliflower, broken into bite-sized pieces
- 1 cup mustard
- 2 Tbsp butter grass-fed
- Salt to taste

Ingredients

1. Combine together almond flour, salt, garlic and half cup water.
2. Put in cauliflower, being sure that all the pieces are coated well.
3. Place cauliflower on a baking sheet in a single layer (use parchment paper or oil to prevent it from sticking).
4. Line the bottom of your Crock Pot with parchment paper and place coated cauliflower.
5. In a small bowl, mix together the mustard and butter.
6. Pour the mustard and butter mixture over the cauliflower.
7. Cover and cook for about 4 hours, until tender.
8. Remove from the Crock Pot and serve.

Note: You can add some herbs to mustard and butter mixture for more intensive taste.

Servings: 4

Cooking Times

Total Time: 4 hours and 10 minutes

Nutrition Facts

Serving size: 1/4 of a recipe (9.5 ounces)

Percent daily values based on the Reference Daily Intake (RDI) for a 2000 calorie diet.

Nutrition information calculated from recipe ingredients.

Amount Per Serving

Calories 114,47

Calories From Fat (52%) 60,08

% Daily Value

Total Fat 6,86g 11%

Saturated Fat 2,06g 10%

Cholesterol 6,16mg 2%

Sodium 241,83mg 10%

Potassium 656,59mg 19%

Total Carbohydrates 11,59g 4%

Fiber 4,75g 19%

Sugar 4,15g

Protein 4,84g 10%

Simple "Baked" Asparagus with Lemon Juice (Crock Pot)

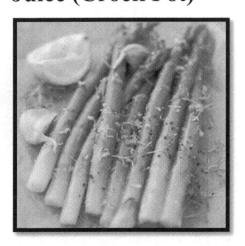

Ingredients

- 1 bunch of fresh asparagus
- 2 cloves minced garlic
- 2 Tbsp butter grass-fed
- Salt and ground pepper to taste
- 1 Lemon juice for serving

Instructions

1. Wash and clean the asparagus: trim the woody end off each asparagus.
2. Line your Crock Pot bowl with baking paper and lay asparagus on paper.
3. Add butter, garlic and salt and pepper to taste.
4. Cook on LOW for 2 hours.

5. Sprinkle with lemon juice and serve.

Servings: 4

Cooking Times

Total Time: 2 hours and 10 minutes

Nutrition Facts

Serving size: 1/4 of a recipe (4 ounces)

Percent daily values based on the Reference Daily Intake (RDI) for a 2000 calorie diet.

Nutrition information calculated from recipe ingredients.

Amount Per Serving

Calories 64,39

Calories From Fat (80%) 51,39

% Daily Value

Total Fat 5,85g 9%

Saturated Fat 3,67g 18%

Cholesterol 15,27mg 5%

Sodium 1,98mg <1%

Potassium 103,74mg 3%

Total Carbohydrates 3,07g 1%

Fiber 0,92g 4%

Sugar 1,14g

Protein 1,09g 2%

BREAKFAST

Breakfast Keto Egg Muffins (Crock Pot)

Ingredients

- 3 green onions (chopped)
- 2 cloves garlic minced
- 1 cup Parmesan, shredded
- 12 eggs
- 1 tsp of Italian seasonings
- Salt and freshly black pepper to taste

Instructions

1. Combine the garlic and the green onions with a pinch of salt.
2. Divide the mixture evenly into the bottom of greased baking muffin cups.
3. Sprinkle Parmesan cheese into each baking cup, over the vegetables.
4. Place the baking cups/paper cups at the bottom of your Crock Pot.
5. Whisk the eggs in mixing bowl with salt, pepper, Italian seasoning.
6. Pour the egg mixture into each baking cups, over the cheese.

7. Cover and cook on HIGH for 2 - 3 hours.

8. Serve hot.

Servings: 12

Cooking Times

Total Time: 3 hours and 10 minutes

Nutrition Facts

Serving size: 1/12 of a recipe (2.5 ounces)

Percent daily values based on the Reference Daily Intake (RDI) for a 2000 calorie diet.

Nutrition information calculated from recipe ingredients.

Amount Per Serving

Calories 111,69

Calories From Fat (63%) 70,42

% Daily Value

Total Fat 7,89g 12%

Saturated Fat 3,55g 18%

Cholesterol 195,89mg 65%

Total Carbohydrates 0,99g <1%

Fiber 0,13g <1%

Sugar 0,33g

Protein 8,74g 17%

Breakfast Piquant Eggs (Crock Pot)

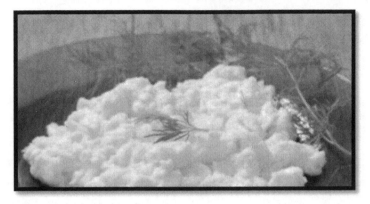

Ingredients

- 2 Tbps of olive oil
- 2 green onion sliced
- 2 pinch grated hot pepper (or to taste)
- 1 tsp cumin
- 8 eggs
- Salt to taste

Instructions

1. Heat the olive oil in a frying pan, and sauté the green onions for 2 - 3 minutes.
2. Season salt, hot pepper, and the cumin.
3. Transfer the onion to your greased Crock Pot.
4. Whisk the eggs with a pinch of salt and extra hot pepper if needed.

5. Pour the egg mixture over the green onions in your Crock Pot.
6. Cover and cook on HIGH for 2 hours.
7. Sprinkle with chopped parsley or dill and serve hot.

Servings: 4

Cooking Times

Total Time: 2 hours and 10 minutes

Nutrition Facts

Serving size: 1/4 of a recipe (6 ounces)

Percent daily values based on the Reference Daily Intake (RDI) for a 2000 calorie diet.

Nutrition information calculated from recipe ingredients.

Amount Per Serving

Calories 230,09

Calories From Fat (64%) 146,94

% Daily Value

Total Fat 16,45g 25%

Saturated Fat 4,1g 21%

Cholesterol 372mg 124%

Total Carbohydrates 6,92g 2%

Fiber 1,2g 5%

Sugar 2,98g

Protein 13,37g 27%

Egg Whites Vegetable Omelet (Crock Pot)

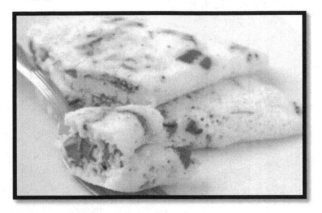

Ingredients

- 2 Tbsp lard or butter
- 1 1/2 cups spinach cooked, drained and chopped
- 1 green onion, minced
- 8 egg whites, beaten
- 1/2 cup Parmesan cheese (grated)
- Salt and pepper, to taste

Instructions

1. Heat the lard in a frying skillet over medium heat.
2. Add the green onion and sauté for 2 - 3 minutes.
3. Add the spinach and sauté for about 3-4 minutes; season salt and pepper.
4. Transfer mixture to your oiled Crock Pot.
5. Whisk the eggs with salt and pepper in a bowl.

6. Pour the egg mixture over spinach and sprinkle generously with Parmesan cheese.
7. Cover and cook on HIGH for about 2 hours.
8. Serve hot.

Servings: 4

Cooking Times

Total Time: 20 minutes

Nutrition Facts

Serving size: 1/4 of a recipe (5.5 ounces)

Percent daily values based on the Reference Daily Intake (RDI) for a 2000 calorie diet.

Nutrition information calculated from recipe ingredients.

Amount Per Serving

Calories 164,49

Calories From Fat (52%) 86,04

% Daily Value

Total Fat 9,81g 15%

Saturated Fat 5,84g 29%

Cholesterol 26,27mg 9%

Total Carbohydrates 5,65g 2%

Fiber 1,91g 8%

Sugar 2,08g

Protein 13,99g 28%

Egg-whites with Cremini Mushrooms Omelet (Crock Pot)

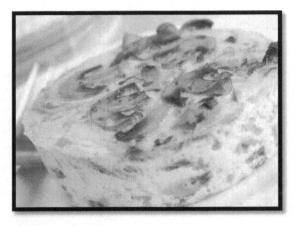

Ingredients

- 12 egg whites
- 2 cups Cremini mushrooms cleaned, sliced
- 3/4 cup Parmesan cheese freshly grated
- 2 Tbsp olive oil
- Salt and ground white pepper to taste

Instructions

1. Whisk the egg whites with salt and pepper until set.
2. Add sliced mushrooms and Parmesan cheese; stir well.
3. Oil your Crock Pot and pour the egg whites mixture.
4. Cover and cook on HIGH for about 2 hours. Omelet is done when eggs are set.
5. Serve hot.

Servings: 4

Cooking Times

Total Time: 15 minutes

Nutrition Facts

Serving size: 1/4 of a recipe (6 ounces)

Percent daily values based on the Reference Daily Intake (RDI) for a 2000 calorie diet.

Nutrition information calculated from recipe ingredients.

Amount Per Serving

Calories 160,51

Calories From Fat (43%) 69,53

% Daily Value

Total Fat 7,9g 12%

Saturated Fat 3,57g 18%

Cholesterol 16,5mg 6%

Sodium 454,81mg 19%

Potassium 298,09mg 9%

Total Carbohydrates 2,63g <1%

Fiber 0,35g 1%

Sugar 1,57g

Protein 19,21g 38%

Flourless Zucchini Quiche with Parmesan Cheese (Crock Pot)

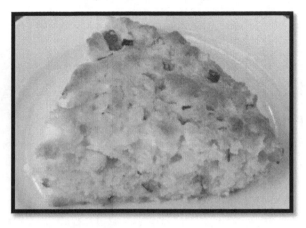

Ingredients

- 1 1/2 lbs of zucchini grated
- 4 eggs preferably organic
- 3 cups Parmesan cheese grated
- 1 cup Greek yogurt (plain and unsweetened)
- 1/2 cup olive oil
- Salt, pepper, fresh mint chopped

Instructions

1. In a large bowl stir zucchini, eggs, cheese, oil, yogurt, mint, salt, and pepper.
2. Cover the bottom of your Slow Cooker with parchment paper and spread the mixture.
3. Sprinkle some more cheese on the top.

29

4. Cover and cook on HIGH for 1 1/2 - 2 hours.

5. Let cool, and serve warm.

Servings: 8

Cooking Times

Total Time: 2 hours and 10 minutes

Nutrition Facts

Serving size: 1/8 of a recipe (8 ounces)

Percent daily values based on the Reference Daily Intake (RDI) for a 2000 calorie diet.

Nutrition information calculated from recipe ingredients.

Amount Per Serving

Calories 336,81

Calories From Fat (77%) 258,21

% Daily Value

Total Fat 29,25g 45%

Saturated Fat 10,38g 52%

Cholesterol 137,55mg 46%

Sodium 178,65mg 7%

Potassium 289,42mg 8%

Total Carbohydrates 2,97g <1%

Fiber 0,85g 3%

Sugar 2,36g

Protein 16,24g 32%

Keto Vegetable Soufflé (Crock Pot)

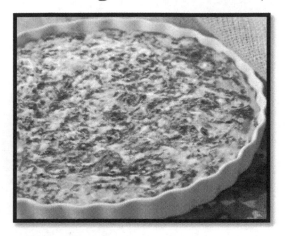

Ingredients

- 2 Tbsp olive oil
- 2 cups fresh spinach chopped
- 1 scallion finely chopped
- 1/4 cup fresh basil (chopped)
- 8 eggs preferably organic
- Sea salt and freshly ground pepper to taste

Instructions

1. Grease your Crock Pot with oil.
2. Layer the spinach, scallion and fresh basil on the bottom of your Crock Pot.
3. Whisk the eggs with salt and pepper in a bowl.
4. Pour the egg mixture over the vegetables.

5. Cover and cook on LOW for about 4-6 hours or on HIGH for 2 hours.
6. When ready, let cool for 5-10 minutes.
7. Serve warm.

Servings: 4

Nutrition Facts

Serving size: 1/4 of a recipe (4 ounces)

Percent daily values based on the Reference Daily Intake (RDI) for a 2000 calorie diet.

Nutrition information calculated from recipe ingredients.

Amount Per Serving

Calories 190,87

Calories From Fat (71%) 135,7

% Daily Value

Total Fat 15,2g 23%

Saturated Fat 3,7g 19%

Cholesterol 327,36mg 109%

Sodium 137,78mg 6%

Potassium 223,39mg 6%

Total Carbohydrates 1,6g <1%

Fiber 0,54g 2%

Sugar 0,48g

Protein 11,62g 23%

Radish Greens and Mushrooms Omelet (Crock Pot)

Instructions

- 1/4 cup olive oil
- 2 cups Radish greens chopped
- 3 cups mushrooms, sliced
- 8 eggs lightly beaten
- 1 cup Cheddar cheese, grated
- Salt and ground black pepper to taste

Instructions

1. Wash the radish greens in cold water. Change the water until any grit or dirt appears, which will settle on the bottom of the sink. Drain the radish greens in a colander.
2. Place the greens and mushrooms on the bottom of your oiled Crock Pot.
3. Whisk the eggs with salt, and pepper and Cheddar cheese until combine well.
4. Pour the egg mixture in Crock Pot.
5. Cover and cook on LOW for 4 - 6 hours.
6. Serve hot.

Servings: 4

Cooking Times

Total Time: 6 hours

Nutrition Facts

Serving size: 1/4 of a recipe (7 ounces)

Percent daily values based on the Reference Daily Intake (RDI) for a 2000 calorie diet.

Nutrition information calculated from recipe ingredients.

Amount Per Serving

Calories 360,7

Calories From Fat (75%) 268,77

% Daily Value

Total Fat 30,32g 47%

Saturated Fat 10,23g 51%

Cholesterol 312,38mg 104%

Sodium 293,25mg 12%

Potassium 398,77mg 11%

Total Carbohydrates 3,99g 1%

Fiber 1,45g 6%

Sugar 1,92g

Protein 18,96g 38%

Savory Kale Patties (Crock Pot)

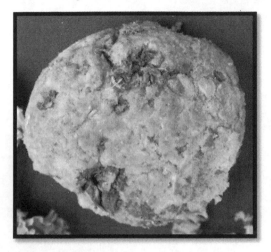

Ingredients

- 1/4 cup olive oil
- 1 cup almond flour
- 1 bunch of kale leaves
- 1/4 tsp red chili powder
- 1/4 tsp turmeric powder
- Black salt or salt as per taste

Instructions

1. In a bowl, mix all the ingredients together.
2. With your wet hands knead the batter with your and shape a kale patties.
3. Oil the inner side of your Crock Pot and layer kale patties one by one.
4. Cover and cook on HIGH for 2-3 hours.

5. Serve immediately.

Servings: 4
Cooking Times
Total Time: 3 hours and 10 minutes
Nutrition Facts
Serving size: 1/4 of a recipe (5 ounces)
Percent daily values based on the Reference Daily Intake (RDI) for a 2000 calorie diet.
Nutrition information calculated from recipe ingredients.
Amount Per Serving
Calories 237,82
Calories From Fat (52%) 123,85
% Daily Value
Total Fat 14,04g 22%
Saturated Fat 2g 10%
Cholesterol 0mg 0%
Sodium 207,28mg 9%
Potassium 347,91mg 10%
Total Carbohydrates 21,4g 7%
Fiber 7,69g 31%
Sugar 0,15g
Protein 7,9g 16%

Spicy Deviled Egg Breakfast (Crock Pot)

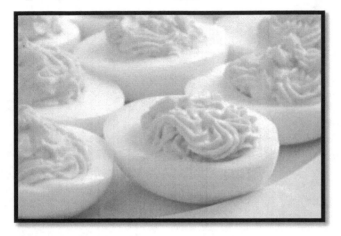

Ingredients

- 8 large eggs preferably organic
- 1/4 cup cream cheese, softened
- 1/2 cup mayonnaise
- 1/4 tsp smoked paprika
- Salt and ground pepper to taste

Instructions

1. Place whole eggs in your Crock and fill with enough water to completely cover eggs.
2. Cook on LOW for 3 1/2 hours.
3. When ready, peel the eggs and slice in half lengthwise.
4. Remove yolks and fork mash them in a medium mixing bowl.
5. Add cream cheese, mayonnaise, and paprika.

6. Stir until all ingredients are well incorporated.
7. Fill the egg halves with mayonnaise mixture.
8. Sprinkle with paprika and refrigerate for one hour.
9. Serve.

Servings: 6
Cooking Times
Total Time: 3 hours and 20 minutes
Nutrition Facts
Serving size: 1/6 of a recipe (4 ounces)
Percent daily values based on the Reference Daily Intake (RDI) for a 2000 calorie diet.
Nutrition information calculated from recipe ingredients.
Amount Per Serving
Calories 205,04
Calories From Fat (70%) 144,13
% Daily Value
Total Fat 16,2g 25%
Saturated Fat 4,91g 25%
Cholesterol 263,73mg 88%
Total Carbohydrates 4,61g 2%
Fiber 0,03g <1%
Sugar 1,82g
Protein 9,14g 18%

Zucchini with Double Cheese Omelet (Crock Pot)

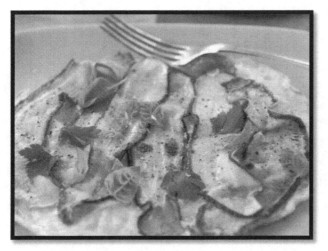

Ingredients

- 4 zucchini sliced
- 3 Tbsp dill finely chopped
- 12 eggs
- 1 cup Cottage cheese
- 3/4 cup Parmesan cheese freshly grated
- Salt and ground pepper to taste

Instructions

1. Grease your Crock Pot and layer sliced zucchini and dill; season with little salt.
2. Whisk the eggs and pour over the zucchini.
3. Sprinkle both kinds of cheese and give a good stir.

4. Cover and cook on HIGH for 2 hours. Omelet is done when eggs are set.
5. Let cool for 10 minutes and serve.

Servings: 6
Cooking Times
Total Time: 2 hours and 15 minutes
Nutrition Facts
Serving size: 1/6 of a recipe (9 ounces)
Percent daily values based on the Reference Daily Intake (RDI) for a 2000 calorie diet.
Nutrition information calculated from recipe ingredients.
Amount Per Serving
Calories 260,11
Calories From Fat (58%) 150,9
% Daily Value
Total Fat 17,01g 26%
Saturated Fat 8,25g 41%
Cholesterol 310,48mg 103%
Total Carbohydrates 6,33g 2%
Fiber 1,59g 6%
Sugar 3,93g
Protein 20,94g 42%

LUNCH

Braised Zoodles, Spinach and Olives (Crock Pot)

Ingredients

- 2 Tbsp ghee
- 2 cup spinach, packed
- 3 large zucchini, spiral sliced
- 12 Kalamata olives halved
- 3/4 cup Parmesan cheese, shredded
- sea salt and black pepper, to taste

Instructions

1. Wash the zucchini under cold water. With the help of mandolin slicer or a regular peeler slice the zucchini and make zoodles.
2. Place ghee on the bottom of your Crock Pot.
3. In a large bowl, combine chopped spinach, zoodles, halved Kalamata olives, sea salt, and black pepper.
4. Toss to combine well and dump in your Crock Pot.
5. Cover and cook on HIGH for 1 - 2 hours or on LOW 3 - 4 hours.
6. Transfer to a serving plate, generously sprinkle with Parmesan and serve.

Servings: 4

Cooking Times

Total Time: 4 hours and 10 minutes

Nutrition Facts

Serving size: 1/4 of a recipe (8 ounces)

Percent daily values based on the Reference Daily Intake (RDI) for a 2000 calorie diet.

Nutrition information calculated from recipe ingredients.

Amount Per Serving

Calories 142,05

Calories From Fat (56%) 78,91

% Daily Value

Total Fat 8,92g 14%

Saturated Fat 3,39g 17%

Cholesterol 16,5mg 6%

Sodium 495,55mg 21%

Potassium 552,88mg 16%

Total Carbohydrates 7,11g 2%

Fiber 2,04g 8%

Sugar 4,13g

Protein 9,73g 19%

Lemony Green Beans (Crock Pot)

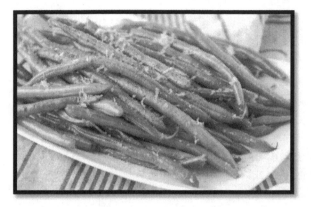

Ingredients

- 1 Tbsp lard or ghee
- 2 lbs of fresh green beans, stem ends trimmed
- 2 Tbsp Apple vinaigrette dressing (or your favorite)
- Juice of 1/2 lemon
- Salt and pepper to taste
- Peel of 1/2 lemon

Instructions

1. Wash and trim the beans. Soak them in a clean sink or bowl filled with and place in a colander.
2. Dump lard or ghee on the bottom of your Crock Pot.
3. Place the green beans and season salt and pepper to taste.
4. Pour the vinaigrette dressing and some water.
5. Cover and cook on HIGH 3 hours or on LOW 4 -5 hours, or until beans are tender.

6. Remove from the heat, cover with foil and let rest for 10 minutes.
7. Pour lemon juice, sprinkle with the lemon zest and serve.

Servings: 4

Cooking Times

Inactive Time: 10 minutes

Total Time: 5 hours and 10 minutes

Nutrition Facts

Serving size: 1/4 of a recipe (9 ounces)

Percent daily values based on the Reference Daily Intake (RDI) for a 2000 calorie diet.

Nutrition information calculated from recipe ingredients.

Amount Per Serving

Calories 74,31

Calories From Fat (7%) 5,02

% Daily Value

Total Fat 0,66g 1%

Saturated Fat 0,14g <1%

Cholesterol 0mg 0%

Total Carbohydrates 17,02g 6%

Fiber 6,23g 25%

Sugar 7,77g

Protein 4,19g 8%

Herbed Portobello Mushrooms (Crock Pot)

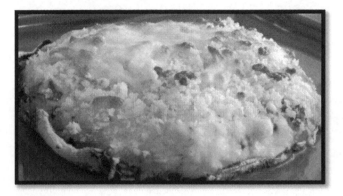

Ingredients

- 1 1/4 lbs Portobello mushrooms
- 2 Tbsp garlic-infused ghee
- 2 Tbsp fresh basil finely chopped
- 1 Tbsp fresh parsley finely chopped
- 2 cups Parmesan cheese, grated
- Salt and pepper to taste

Instructions

1. Clean and slice the mushrooms.
2. Heat the ghee in a non-stick frying pan over medium heat.
3. Add the sliced mushrooms, season with salt and pepper and cook for about 5 minutes.
4. Transfer the mushrooms in your Crock Pot.
5. Wash and finely chop your basil and parsley.

6. Sprinkle herbs over the mushrooms and top with grated parmesan cheese.
7. Cover the lid and cook on HIGH for about 3 hours or until the mushroom is cooked through.
8. Serve hot.

Servings: 4
Cooking Times
Total Time: 3 hours and 10 minutes
Nutrition Facts
Serving size: 1/4 of a recipe (7.5 ounces)
Percent daily values based on the Reference Daily Intake (RDI) for a 2000 calorie diet.
Nutrition information calculated from recipe ingredients.
Amount Per Serving
Calories 252,27
Calories From Fat (52%) 130,43
% Daily Value
Total Fat 14,89g 23%
Saturated Fat 8,77g 44%
Total Carbohydrates 6,79g 3%
Fiber 2,3g 9%
Sugar 3,3g
Protein 24,16g 48%

Button Mushrooms with Herbs de Provence (Crock Pot)

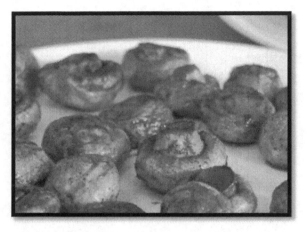

Ingredients

- 1 lb button mushrooms, stems removed
- 1 Tbsp Herbs de Provence
- 1/4 cup Extra virgin olive oil
- 1/2 tsp mild pepper flakes
- Sea salt and black pepper to taste

Instructions

1. In a bowl, mix Herbs de Provence, olive oil, pepper flakes, salt and pepper to taste.
2. Wash and clean the mushrooms, and dry on paper towel.
3. Rub the mushrooms all over with herbs mixture.
4. Pour olive oil on the bottom of your Crock Pot and arrange the mushrooms with cups down.

5. Cover and cook on HIGH for about 3 hours or until the mushroom is cooked through.
6. Serve and enjoy!

Servings: 6
Cooking Times
Total Time: 3 hours and 10 minutes
Nutrition Facts
Serving size: 1/6 of a recipe (12 ounces)
Percent daily values based on the Reference Daily Intake (RDI) for a 2000 calorie diet.
Nutrition information calculated from recipe ingredients.
Amount Per Serving
Calories 167,67
Calories From Fat (53%) 89,1
% Daily Value
Total Fat 10,14g 16%
Saturated Fat 1,44g 7%
Cholesterol 0mg 0%
Sodium 30,29mg 1%
Total Carbohydrates 7,11g 4%
Fiber 4,24g 17%
Sugar 8,17g
Protein 6,83g 14%

Simple Lemony-Garlic Artichokes (Crock Pot)

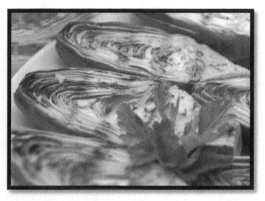

Ingredients

- 4 artichokes
- 3 cloves of garlic minced
- 3 Tbsp lemon juice (freshly squeezed)
- 1/2 cup of extra virgin olive oil
- 3 fresh sprigs of parsley finely chopped
- Sea salt

Instructions

1. Wash the artichokes, and then clean the outer leaves.
2. Using a knife cut off the top of the artichoke and trim the very bottom of the stem.
3. Place trimmed artichokes in your Crock Pot.
4. Season each artichoke with salt and pepper.

5. Place minced garlic on top of each artichoke and drizzle olive oil evenly over each artichoke top.
6. Pour the lemon juice and olive oil.
7. Cover the lid and cook on HIGH for 3-4 hours.
8. Decorate with freshly chopped parsley leaves and serve hot.

Servings: 5

Cooking Times

Total Time: 4 hours and 10 minutes

Nutrition Facts

Serving size: 1/5 of a recipe (6 ounces)

Percent daily values based on the Reference Daily Intake (RDI) for a 2000 calorie diet.

Nutrition information calculated from recipe ingredients.

Amount Per Serving

Calories 65,72

Calories From Fat (3%) 1,92

% Daily Value

Total Fat 0,23g <1%

Saturated Fat 0,05g <1%

Total Carbohydrates 14,87g 5%

Fiber 7,07g 28%

Sugar 1,53g

Protein 4,39g 9%

Zucchini and Shiitake "Stew" (Crock Pot)

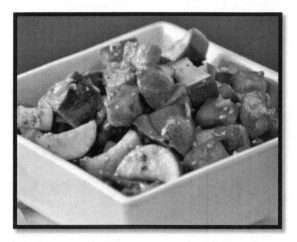

Ingredients

- 1 Tbsp lard
- 4 zucchini sliced
- 3 cups Shiitake mushrooms, sliced
- 1 scallion chopped
- 4 sprigs fresh rosemary chopped
- Sea salt and freshly ground black pepper to taste

Instructions

1. In a large mixing bowl, combine zucchini, mushrooms, scallion, chopped rosemary, sea salt, and black pepper. Toss until vegetables are coated and ingredients are well mixed.
2. Pour half cup water and cover.
3. Cook on HIGH for 2 - 3 hours or on LOW for 4 - 5 hours.

4. Taste and adjust salt and pepper to taste.
5. Serve hot.

Servings: 4
Cooking Times
Total Time: 5 hours and 10 minutes
Nutrition Facts
Serving size: 1/4 of a recipe (10 ounces)
Percent daily values based on the Reference Daily Intake (RDI) for a 2000 calorie diet.
Nutrition information calculated from recipe ingredients.
Amount Per Serving
Calories 96,09
Calories From Fat (39%) 37,54
% Daily Value
Total Fat 4,23g 7%
Saturated Fat 1,3g 7%
Cholesterol 3,04mg 1%
Sodium 17,94mg <1%
Potassium 592,14mg 17%
Total Carbohydrates 13,37g 4%
Fiber 5,03g 20%
Sugar 4,55g
Protein 4,33g 9%

DINNER

"Baked" Broccoli with Lemon and Parmesan (Crock Pot)

Ingredients

- 4 cups broccoli florets, cut into small pieces
- 1/4 cup virgin olive oil
- 1/2 lemon zest
- 1 1/2 tsp lemon juice, freshly squeezed
- 4 Tbsp freshly ground Parmesan Cheese
- Salt and pepper to taste

Instructions

1. Wash, clean and chop broccoli into small pieces.
2. Place broccoli pieces in your Crock Pot.
3. Pour water, oil, and lemon zest, lemon juice into Crock Pot with broccoli.
4. Sprinkle salt and black pepper on top of the broccoli.
5. Close lid and cook on LOW for 2-3 hours.
6. Transfer broccoli to a platter and sprinkle with grated Parmesan.
7. Serve immediately.

Servings: 4

Cooking Times

Total Time: 3 hours

Nutrition Facts

Serving size: 1/4 of a recipe (4.5 ounces)

Percent daily values based on the Reference Daily Intake (RDI) for a 2000 calorie diet.

Nutrition information calculated from recipe ingredients.

Amount Per Serving

Calories 161,89

Calories From Fat (83%) 133,98

% Daily Value

Total Fat 15,19g 23%

Saturated Fat 2,77g 14%

Cholesterol 4,4mg 1%

Sodium 96mg 4%

Potassium 241,5mg 7%

Total Carbohydrates 4,29g 1%

Fiber 0,16g <1%

Sugar 0,16g

Protein 4,07g 8%

"Roasted" Cayenne Sweet Potatoes Crock Pot)

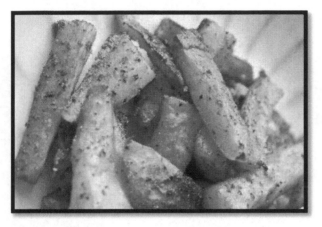

Ingredients

- 4 medium sweet potatoes
- 1 tsp Cayenne pepper, optional
- 1 Tbsp smoked paprika
- 1/4 cup olive oil
- Salt to taste

Instructions

1. Wash the sweet potatoes well; peel them off.
2. Slice the sweet potatoes into wedges.
3. In a bowl, combine the potatoes with the rest of the ingredients from the list.
4. Oil the bottom of your Crock Pot and lay sweet potato wedges.

5. Cover and cook on LOW for about 4 - 4 1/2 hours.
6. Serve hot.

Servings: 4
Cooking Times
Total Time: 4 hours
Nutrition Facts
Serving size: 1/4 of a recipe (5.5 ounces)
Percent daily values based on the Reference Daily Intake (RDI) for a 2000 calorie diet.
Nutrition information calculated from recipe ingredients.
Amount Per Serving
Calories 236,29
Calories From Fat (52%) 121,88
% Daily Value
Total Fat 13,8g 21%
Saturated Fat 1,93g 10%
Cholesterol 0mg 0%
Sodium 72,96mg 3%
Potassium 479,26mg 14%
Total Carbohydrates 27,14g 9%
Fiber 4,52g 18%
Sugar 5,62g
Protein 2,29g 5%

Aromatic Broccoli and Tarragon Soup (Crock Pot)

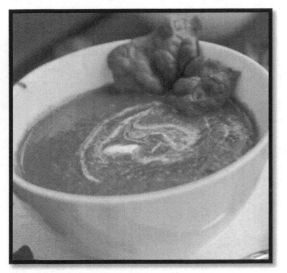

Ingredients

- 1/4 cup Olive oil
- 3 cloves garlic, chopped
- 4 lbs. of broccoli, stems peeled and cut into chunks
- 1 Tbsp fresh tarragon finely chopped
- 4-5 cups water
- Salt and ground black pepper to taste

Instructions

1. In a non-stick frying pan, heat the olive oil over medium heat.

2. Add chopped garlic with a pinch of salt and sauté 2 -3 minutes.
3. Place in broccoli and chopped tarragon, and cover with water.
4. Season salt and pepper.
5. Transfer the broccoli mixture to your Crock Pot and cover.
6. Cook on HIGH for 2 hours or LOW for 4-6 hours, until the broccoli is tender.
7. Transfer the mixture to your blender and blend until smooth.
8. Taste, adjust salt and pepper and serve immediately.

Servings: 6

Cooking Times

Total Time: 6 hours and 5 minutes

Nutrition Facts

Serving size: 1/6 of a recipe (11 ounces)

Percent daily values based on the Reference Daily Intake (RDI) for a 2000 calorie diet.

Nutrition information calculated from recipe ingredients.

Amount Per Serving

Calories 132,01

Calories From Fat (68%) 89,7

% Daily Value

Total Fat 10,23g 16%

Saturated Fat 1,4g 7%

Cholesterol 0mg 0%

Sodium 43,84mg 2%

Potassium 469,96mg 13%

Total Carbohydrates 6,72g 3%

Fiber 0,91g 4%

Sugar 0,01g

Protein 4,65g 9%

Brussels Sprout with Feta Cheese (Crock Pot)

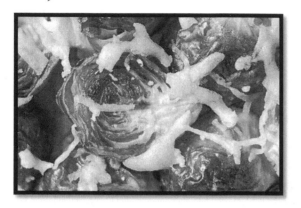

Ingredients

- 14 Brussels sprouts
- 2 cloves garlic
- 1/4 cup Feta cheese crumbled
- 1/2 cup cream cheese
- 1 tsp fresh lemon juice
- Salt and pepper to taste

Instructions

1. Rinse the Brussels sprouts in cold water to remove any dust or dirt. Clean the Brussels and discard first leaves.
2. Grease the bottom of your Crock Pot and lay Brussels sprouts. Add all remaining ingredients and stir well.
3. Cover and cook on LOW heat for 3-4 hours or HIGH heat for 1-2 hours.

4. Before serving, sprinkle with crumbled Feta cheese.

5. Let cheese melt for 2-3 minutes.

6. Serve and enjoy!

Servings: 2

Cooking Times

Total Time: 4 hours and 10 minutes

Nutrition Facts

Serving size: 1/2 of a recipe (7 ounces)

Percent daily values based on the Reference Daily Intake (RDI) for a 2000 calorie diet.

Nutrition information calculated from recipe ingredients.

Amount Per Serving

Calories 222,57

Calories From Fat (64%) 142,92

% Daily Value

Total Fat 16,27g 25%

Saturated Fat 9,59g 48%

Cholesterol 54,97mg 18%

Total Carbohydrates 8,55g 5%

Fiber 4,4g 18%

Sugar 3,49g

Protein 8,78g 18%

Butternut Squash Soup with Herb Blend (Crock Pot)

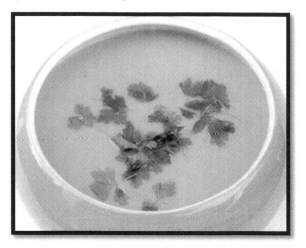

Ingredients

- 1/4 cup olive oil
- 1 1/2 lb diced butternut squash
- 1 1/2 quarts water
- 1 Tbsp Italian Herb Blend
- 2 Tbsp fresh rosemary finely chopped

Instructions

1. First, finely chop the fresh rosemary; set aside.
2. Next, cut the squash in half lengthwise, and slice it crosswise.
3. Cut the squash halves in half again lengthwise, then slice crosswise.

4. Pour the olive in your Crock Pot.
5. Place the squash cubes along with water, Italian Herb Blend and fresh rosemary finely chopped. Stir and cover lid.
6. Cook on HIGH for 2 hours or on LOW for 4 - 5 hours until squash is very tender.
7. When ready, use an immersion blender to puree the mixture.
8. B back soup in your Crock Pot, cover and cook on LOW for 1 hour more.
9. Taste and season salt and fresh-ground black pepper if needed.
10. Serve hot.

Servings: 8
Cooking Times
Total Time: 5 hours and 15 minutes
Nutrition Facts
Serving size: 1/8 of a recipe (9.5 ounces)
Percent daily values based on the Reference Daily Intake (RDI) for a 2000 calorie diet.
Nutrition information calculated from recipe ingredients.
Amount Per Serving
Calories 99,62

Calories From Fat (61%) 60,82

% Daily Value

Total Fat 6,89g 11%

Saturated Fat 0,96g 5%

Cholesterol 0mg 0%

Sodium 9,16mg <1%

Potassium 304,06mg 9%

Total Carbohydrates 7,29g 3%

Fiber 1,84g 7%

Sugar 1,87g

Protein 0,9g 2%

Cauliflower Puree with Sesame (Crock Pot)

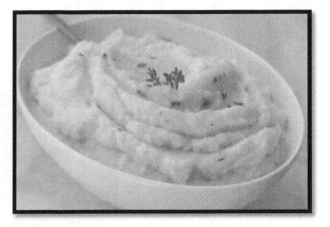

Ingredients

- 1 head cauliflower in florets
- 1 leek finely chopped
- 2 Tbsp butter, unsalted and softened
- 1 cup full-fat cream
- 1 Tbsp sesame seeds toasted
- Salt and ground pepper to taste

Instructions

1. Wash the cauliflower and remove the stem. In this phase, the cauliflower will naturally fall apart into large florets.
2. Break the large florets down into smaller with your knife.
3. Place the cauliflower in your Crock Pot along with finely chopped leek.

4. Season salt and pour enough water to cover completely the vegetables.
5. Cover and cook for HIGH for 2 -3 hours or on LOW for 6 hours.
6. Remove the cauliflower and leeks from the water, and place in your blender.
7. Add the butter, full-fat cream, sesame seeds and blend until soft and creamy.
8. Taste and adjust salt and pepper. Blend for 15 seconds more.
9. Sprinkle with some more sesame seeds and serve immediately.

Servings: 6
Cooking Times
Total Time: 6 hours and 10 minutes
Nutrition Facts
Serving size: 1/6 of a recipe (7 ounces)
Percent daily values based on the Reference Daily Intake (RDI) for a 2000 calorie diet.
Nutrition information calculated from recipe ingredients.
Amount Per Serving
Calories 250,08
Calories From Fat (65%) 162,38

% Daily Value

Total Fat 19,19g 30%

Saturated Fat 4,62g 23%

Cholesterol 10,23mg 3%

Sodium 48,84mg 2%

Potassium 587,02mg 17%

Total Carbohydrates 9,1g 5%

Fiber 6,61g 26%

Sugar 3,35g

Protein 8,27g 17%

Creamy Spinach-Chard Soup (Crock Pot)

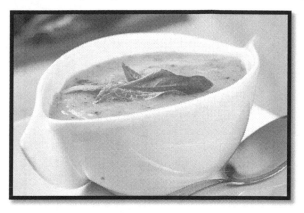

Ingredients

- 1 lb baby spinach leaves
- 1/2 lb Swiss chard, tender stems and leaves finely chopped
- 2 leeks finely chopped
- 1/4 cup extra-virgin olive oil
- 3 cups water
- Salt and black ground pepper to taste

Instructions

1. Heat the olive oil in a non-stick frying pan over medium heat.
2. Sauté the leek for about 2-3 minutes.
3. Add the chard and spinach leaves and stir well.
4. Pour water and season with salt and pepper to taste.
5. Pour the mixture into your oiled Crock Pot.

6. Cover and cook on LOW for 3 hours.
7. Transfer soup to your fast-speed blender and blend until soft completely.
8. Taste, adjust salt and pepper to taste and serve. (you can serve it with fresh lemon juice)

Servings: 6
Cooking Times
Total Time: 3 hours
Nutrition Facts
Serving size: 1/6 of a recipe (10 ounces)
Percent daily values based on the Reference Daily Intake (RDI) for a 2000 calorie diet.
Nutrition information calculated from recipe ingredients.
Amount Per Serving
Calories 44,45
Calories From Fat (9%) 4,06
% Daily Value
Total Fat 0,49g <1%
Saturated Fat 0,08g <1%
Total Carbohydrates 6,64g 3%
Fiber 2,97g 12%
Sugar 1,92g
Protein 3,51g 7%

Light Vegetable Soup (Crock Pot)

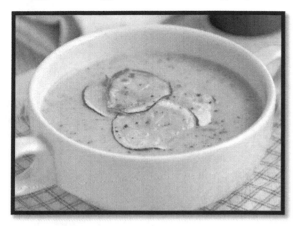

Ingredients

- 1 green onion, diced
- 2 zucchini, sliced
- 2 medium turnips chopped
- 1 cup broccoli florets
- 2 cups water
- salt and black ground pepper to taste

Instructions

1. Place all ingredients from the list (except zucchini) in your Crock Pot.
2. Cook on LOW for 6 hours.
3. When ready, add the chopped zucchini, cover the lid and cook 1 hour on LOW mode.
4. Transfer soup to a blender and blend until smooth well.

5. Taste, adjust salt and pepper and serve hot.

Servings: 4

Cooking Times
Total Time: 7 hours

Nutrition Facts
Serving size: 1/4 of a recipe (11 ounces)
Percent daily values based on the Reference Daily Intake (RDI) for a 2000 calorie diet.
Nutrition information calculated from recipe ingredients.
Amount Per Serving
Calories 49,33
Calories From Fat (8%) 4,14
% Daily Value
Total Fat 0,49g <1%
Saturated Fat 0,11g <1%
Cholesterol 0mg 0%
Total Carbohydrates 10,3g 3%
Fiber 2,78g 11%
Sugar 6,14g
Protein 2,67g 5%

Beetroot and Fresh Mint Salad (Crock Pot)

Ingredients

- 1 lb beetroot
- 2 Tbsp fresh lemon juice (about 2 lemons)
- 3 Tbs of olive oil
- 2/3 cup of fresh mint finely chopped
- 2 spring onions, sliced
- salt and pepper to taste

Instructions

1. Wash well your beets.
2. Place the beets in a Crock Pot and add water (to completely cover beets) and the lemon juice.
3. Cover and cook for 6 hours on LOW or until tender.
4. Rinse, wash and peel the beets.
5. Cut beets into cubes and place in a colander to drain well. Cover and refrigerate for 2-3 hours.
6. Whisk the olive oil with the lemon juice, spring onion and half of mint.
7. Pour the dressing over the beetroot cubes.
8. Add remaining mint and lightly stir.
9. Taste, season salt, and pepper to taste and serve.

Servings: 4

Cooking Times

Inactive Time: 3 hours

Total Time: 6 hours and 20 minutes

Nutrition Facts

Serving size: 1/4 of a recipe (6 ounces)

Percent daily values based on the Reference Daily Intake (RDI) for a 2000 calorie diet.

Nutrition information calculated from recipe ingredients.

Amount Per Serving

Calories 152,21

Calories From Fat (60%) 91,93

% Daily Value

Total Fat 10,41g 16%

Saturated Fat 1,45g 7%

Cholesterol 0mg 0%

Sodium 90,83mg 4%

Potassium 411,41mg 12%

Total Carbohydrates 10,14g 5%

Fiber 3,82g 15%

Sugar 5,87g

Protein 2,27g 5%

Braised Mushrooms and Sage Mash (Crock Pot)

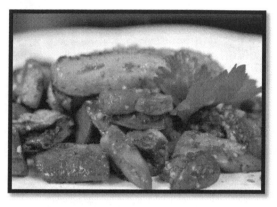

Instructions

- 2 Tbsp olive oil
- 2 cloves garlic minced
- 4 cups mushrooms, thinly sliced
- 2 Tbsp sliced fresh sage, packed
- 1/4 cup water
- Salt and black ground pepper to taste

Instructions

1. Heat the olive oil in medium skillet over medium heat.
2. Add garlic and sauté for 1 minute.
3. Add the mushrooms and sage and sauté for about 5 minutes.
4. Place the mushrooms and sage mixture in your Crock Pot.

5. Cover and cook on LOW heat for 3-4 hours or HIGH heat for 1-2 hours.
6. Serve hot.

Servings: 4

Cooking Times
Total Time: 4 hours

Nutrition Facts
Serving size: 1/4 of a recipe (6 ounces)
Percent daily values based on the Reference Daily Intake (RDI) for a 2000 calorie diet.
Nutrition information calculated from recipe ingredients.
Amount Per Serving
Calories 79,94
Calories From Fat (42%) 33,59
% Daily Value
Total Fat 3,83g 6%
Saturated Fat 0,58g 3%
Total Carbohydrates 3,91g 2%
Fiber 1,37g 5%
Sugar 2,16g
Protein 3,11g 6%

"Roasted" Green Beans with Parmesan (Crock Pot)

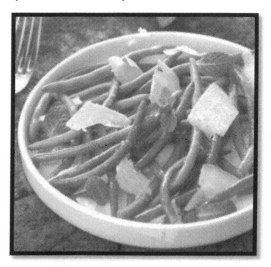

Ingredients

- 2 lbs. fresh green beans, trimmed
- 2 – 3 Tbsp olive oil
- 1 tsp kosher salt and black pepper
- 1/2 cup Parmesan cheese, grated

Instructions

1. Rinse the green beans and dry with paper towels.
2. Drizzle with olive oil and sprinkle with salt and pepper.
3. Use your hands to coat green beans evenly with olive oil.
4. Place green beans in your greased Crock Pot.
5. Generously sprinkle with Parmesan cheese.

6. Cover and cook on HIGH heat setting for 3-4 hours.

7. Serve hot or cold.

Servings: 8

Cooking Times

Total Time: 4 hours and 5 minutes

Nutrition Facts

Serving size: 1/8 of a recipe (5.5 ounces)

Percent daily values based on the Reference Daily Intake (RDI) for a 2000 calorie diet.

Nutrition information calculated from recipe ingredients.

Amount Per Serving

Calories 91,93

Calories From Fat (52%) 47,61

% Daily Value

Total Fat 5,41g 8%

Saturated Fat 1,6g 8%

Cholesterol 5,5mg 2%

Sodium 337,43mg 14%

Potassium 247,12mg 7%

Total Carbohydrates 8,16g 3%

Fiber 3,06g 12%

Sugar 3,75g

Protein 4,48g 9%

Sour Creamy Spinach Soup (Crock Pot)

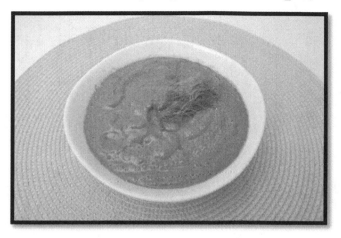

Ingredients

2 Tbs of olive oil

2 spring onions, sliced

1 lb fresh spinach (or frozen)

1/4 cup lemon, juice

1 can (11 oz) Coconut milk

4 cups of water

Instructions

1) Heat the oil in a frying pan over medium heat.

2) Sauté sliced green onions with a pinch of salt for 3 - 4 minutes until soft.

3) Add the spinach and stir well; sauté for 2-3 minutes.

4) Transfer the spinach mixture to your Crock Pot, pour 4 cups of water, lemon juice, and season salt.

5) Close the lid and cook on HIGH for 3-4 hours.
6) When ready, transfer soup to a blender and add coconut milk; blend until creamy.
7) Taste and adjust salt and lemon juice to taste.
8) Serve.

Servings: 6
Cooking Times
Total Time: 4 hours and 10 minutes
Nutrition Facts
Serving size: 1/6 of a recipe (10.5 ounces)
Percent daily values based on the Reference Daily Intake (RDI) for a 2000 calorie diet.
Nutrition information calculated from recipe ingredients.
Amount Per Serving
Calories 141,96
Calories From Fat (79%) 112,12
% Daily Value
Total Fat 13,16g 20%
Saturated Fat 8,05g 40%
Total Carbohydrates 5,81g 2%
Fiber 1,98g 8%
Sugar 0,53g
Protein 3,13g 6%

Zucchini Blossoms Pie (Crock Pot)

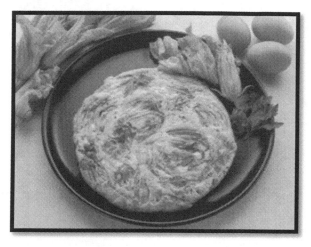

Ingredients

- 2 Tbsp of butter, grass-fed
- ¾ lb zucchini flowers (blossom)
- 5-6 fresh mint leaves, finely chopped
- 4 eggs
- 3 cups grated Cheddar cheese (or Parmesan)
- Salt and ground pepper to taste

Instructions

1. Place butter on the bottom of your Slow Cooker.
2. Clean the zucchini flowers from the stalks and wash them.
3. Place the zucchini flowers with mint leaves in the Slow Cooker.
4. Beat the eggs with salt and pepper in a bowl.

5. Pour the egg mixture over zucchini flowers add sprinkle the cheese.
6. Cover and cook on LOW for 2 hours.
7. Slice and serve hot.

Servings: 3

Cooking Times

Total Time: 2 hours

Nutrition Facts

Serving size: 1/3 of a recipe (7 ounces)

Percent daily values based on the Reference Daily Intake (RDI) for a 2000 calorie diet.

Nutrition information calculated from recipe ingredients.

Amount Per Serving

Calories 271,71

Calories From Fat (69%) 187,52

% Daily Value

Total Fat 21,18g 33%

Saturated Fat 11,27g 56%

Cholesterol 290,35mg 97%

Total Carbohydrates 1,66g <1%

Fiber 0,09g <1%

Sugar 0,48g

Protein 18,11g 36%

Zucchini and Feta "Casserole" (Crock Pot)

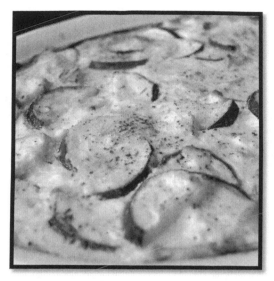

Ingredients

- 4 large zucchinis
- 1 1/2 cup feta cheese
- 1/2 tsp ground onion
- 2 cloves garlic, minced
- 3 eggs
- Salt and pepper to taste

Instructions

1. Slice the zucchinis and place in your Crock Pot.
2. Whisk the eggs along with Feta cheese, chopped or minced garlic, ground onion and salt and pepper.

3. Pour the egg mixture into Slow Cooker over zucchini slices.
4. Cover and cook on HIGH for 3 hours.
5. Let cool for 5 – 10 minutes and serve.

Servings: 6
Cooking Times
Total Time: 3 hours
Nutrition Facts
Serving size: 1/6 of a recipe (10 ounces)
Percent daily values based on the Reference Daily Intake (RDI) for a 2000 calorie diet.
Nutrition information calculated from recipe ingredients.
Amount Per Serving
Calories 171,69
Calories From Fat (57%) 97,55
% Daily Value
Total Fat 11,05g 17%
Saturated Fat 6,57g 33%
Cholesterol 126,28mg 42%
Total Carbohydrates 6,49g 2%
Fiber 2,17g 9%
Sugar 4,04g
Protein 11,08g 22%

Zucchini and Feta "Casserole" (Crock Pot)

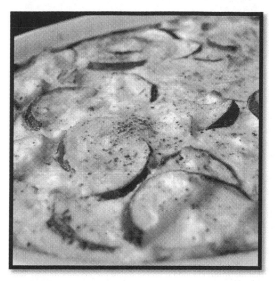

Ingredients

- 4 large zucchinis
- 1 1/2 cup feta cheese
- 1/2 tsp ground onion
- 2 cloves garlic, minced
- 3 eggs
- Salt and pepper to taste

Instructions

1. Slice the zucchinis and place in your Crock Pot.
2. Whisk the eggs along with Feta cheese, chopped or minced garlic, ground onion and salt and pepper.

3. Pour the egg mixture into Slow Cooker over zucchini slices.
4. Cover and cook on HIGH for 3 hours.
5. Let cool for 5 – 10 minutes and serve.

Servings: 6
Cooking Times
Total Time: 3 hours
Nutrition Facts
Serving size: 1/6 of a recipe (10 ounces)
Percent daily values based on the Reference Daily Intake (RDI) for a 2000 calorie diet.
Nutrition information calculated from recipe ingredients.
Amount Per Serving
Calories 171,69
Calories From Fat (57%) 97,55
% Daily Value
Total Fat 11,05g 17%
Saturated Fat 6,57g 33%
Cholesterol 126,38mg 42%
Total Carbohydrates 6,49g 3%
Fiber 2,17g 9%
Sugar 4,04g
Protein 11,08g 22%

SIDE DISH

"Chubby" Spinach Dip (Crock Pot)

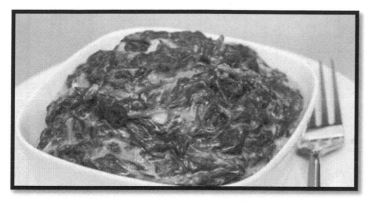

Ingredients

- 1 lb frozen spinach-drained
- 1/2 cup cheese cream
- 3/4 cup Parmesan cheese
- 1/2 cup heavy cream
- 1 clove garlic, minced

Instructions

1. Remove the frozen spinach from the box and place it in a microwave-safe bowl for 1 - 2 minutes.
2. Drain the spinach in a colander.
3. Place all ingredients from the list into your Crock Pot.
4. Cover and cook on HIGH for 2 hours.
5. Give a good stir and serve warm or cold.

Servings: 4

Cooking Times

Total Time: 2 hours and 10 minutes

Nutrition Facts

Serving size: 1/4 of a recipe (7 ounces)

Percent daily values based on the Reference Daily Intake (RDI) for a 2000 calorie diet.

Nutrition information calculated from recipe ingredients.

Amount Per Serving

Calories 277

Calories From Fat (66%) 183,57

% Daily Value

Total Fat 20,94g 32%

Saturated Fat 12,3g 62%

Cholesterol 68,26mg 23%

Sodium 854,39mg 36%

Potassium 406,85mg 12%

Total Carbohydrates 6,79g 3%

Fiber 4,21g 17%

Sugar 0,9g

Protein 17,22g 34%

Broccoli with Nutmeg Dip (Crock Pot)

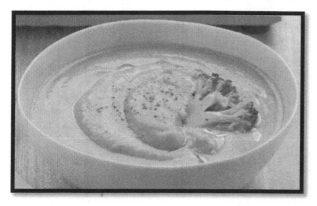

Ingredients

- 1/2 cup of olive oil
- 2 lbs of broccoli
- 1 medium leek (the white part), cut into slices
- 2 tsp nutmeg, grated
- 1 cup of full-fat cream
- Salt and freshly ground pepper

Instructions

1. Cut the main stalk off of fresh broccoli with a sharp knife, and then rinse the broccoli under cool running water. Place the broccoli into your Crock Pot.
2. Chop the leek, only white parts, and sprinkle over the broccoli.
3. Season salt and pepper, and sprinkle with nutmeg.
4. Pour the water enough to cover the broccoli and cover lid.

5. Cook for 2 - 3 hours, or until the broccoli is tender.

6. Transfer broccoli to a blender and pour the cream.

7. Blend until smooth and creamy.

8. Taste and adjust salt and pepper to taste.

9. Serve.

Servings: 8

Cooking Times

Total Time: 3 hours and 5 minutes

Nutrition Facts

Serving size: 1/8 of a recipe (6 ounces)

Percent daily values based on the Reference Daily Intake (RDI) for a 2000 calorie diet.

Nutrition information calculated from recipe ingredients.

Amount Per Serving

Calories 261,47

Calories From Fat (85%) 221,13

% Daily Value

Total Fat 25,11g 39%

Saturated Fat 8,92g 45%

Total Carbohydrates 6,26g 3%

Fiber 0,31g 1%

Sugar 0,62g

Protein 3,98g 8%

Creamy Eggplant Salad with Lemon Juice (Crock Pot)

Ingredients

- 3 medium eggplants whole
- 1 cup full-fat yogurt
- 1 cup fresh basil finely chopped
- 2 Tbsp olive oil
- 2 lemons (zest and lemon juice)
- Salt and freshly ground pepper

Instructions

1. Pierce the eggplant with a knife in different places.
2. Pour one cup water into your Crock Pot and place the eggplants.
3. Cover and cook on LOW for 4 to 6 hours or until eggplant is soft.
4. Remove the eggplant from the pot and let cool for 10 minutes.
5. Peel the skin of eggplant and remove the inner part with a spoon, finely chop and leave for 30 minutes on a strainer to drain off the liquids.
6. Place the eggplant in a large bowl, and add the yogurt, fresh basil, olive oil, lemon juice and lemon zest; stir well.

7. Season salt and pepper to taste and give a good stir.
8. Serve.

Servings: 8
Cooking Times
Inactive Time: 40 minutes
Total Time: 6 hours and 10 minutes
Nutrition Facts
Serving size: 1/8 of a recipe (8 ounces)
Percent daily values based on the Reference Daily Intake (RDI) for a 2000 calorie diet.
Nutrition information calculated from recipe ingredients.
Amount Per Serving
Calories 82,25
Calories From Fat (41%) 34,08
% Daily Value
Total Fat 3,89g 6%
Saturated Fat 0,62g 3%
Cholesterol 0mg 0%
Sodium 7,01mg <1%
Total Carbohydrates 8,18g 4%
Fiber 7,7g 31%
Sugar 4,18g
Protein 2,79g 6%

Hot Artichoke and Double Cheese Mash (Crock Pot)

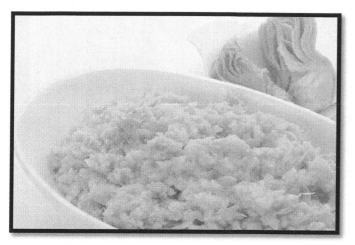

Ingredients

- 2 medium artichoke, chopped
- 1 cup mayonnaise
- 16 oz Mozzarella cheese, shredded
- 1 cup Parmesan cheese freshly grated
- Chopped green onion, optional

Instructions

1. Cut back tough outer leaves of the artichoke until you get down to the yellow leaves.
2. Next, cut off the top third of the artichoke and trim the very bottom of the stem.
3. Using a teaspoon remove the fibrous 'choke' and discard.

4. Cut the artichokes into small pieces.
5. Grease with oil or lard the bottom of your Crock Pot and place the artichokes.
6. Pour the mayonnaise, and sprinkle with Mozzarella and Parmesan cheese.
7. Stir and add two-three tablespoon of water.
8. Cover lid and cook on HIGH for 3-4 hours or on LOW for 5-6 hours.
9. Sprinkle with finely chopped green onion and serve warm.

Servings: 6
Cooking Times
Total Time: 30 minutes
Nutrition Facts
Serving size: 1/6 of a recipe (6.5 ounces)
Percent daily values based on the Reference Daily Intake (RDI) for a 2000 calorie diet.
Nutrition information calculated from recipe ingredients.
Amount Per Serving
Calories 436,66
Calories From Fat (60%) 263,74
% Daily Value
Total Fat 29,95g 46%

Saturated Fat 12,46g 62%

Cholesterol 73,23mg 24%

Sodium 1041,38mg 43%

Potassium 245,73mg 7%

Total Carbohydrates 9,62g 6%

Fiber 2,3g 9%

Sugar 3,93g

Protein 26,5g 53%

Hot Slaw with Blue Cheese (Crock Pot)

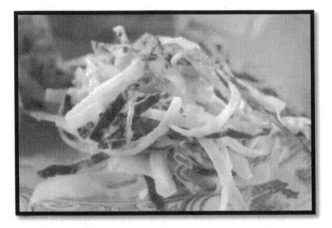

Ingredients

- 1/4 cup olive oil
- 2 lbs cabbage, cut into wedges
- 2 cloves garlic thinly sliced
- 1 Tbsp chopped fresh thyme
- 1/2 cup blue cheese melted (optional)
- Salt and freshly ground black pepper to taste

Instructions

1. Wash and chop the cabbage.
2. Pour the olive oil in your Crock Pot and place the cabbage.
3. Chop finely the garlic and sprinkle over the cabbage.
4. Sprinkle the thyme and season salt and pepper; stir well.
5. Pour one cup of fresh water and stir again.

6. Cover and cook on HIGH for 4 - 6 hours or until cabbage is tender.
7. Taste and adjust the seasonings.
8. Serve hot with melted blue cheese on the top.

Servings: 6
Cooking Times
Total Time: 6 hours
Nutrition Facts
Serving size: 1/6 of a recipe (6.6 ounces)
Percent daily values based on the Reference Daily Intake (RDI) for a 2000 calorie diet.
Nutrition information calculated from recipe ingredients.
Amount Per Serving
Calories 152,61
Calories From Fat (69%) 104,81
% Daily Value
Total Fat 11,88g 18%
Saturated Fat 3,06g 15%
Cholesterol 7,09mg 2%
Total Carbohydrates 6,42g 3%
Fiber 3,86g 15%
Sugar 3,9g
Protein 4,04g 8%

Lemony Shiitake and Broccoli (Crock Pot)

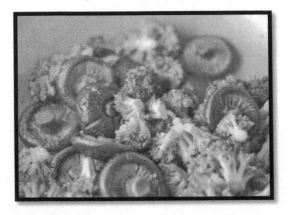

Ingredients

- 2 Tbsp minced garlic
- 2 broccoli heads
- 2 cups mushrooms (chopped fine)
- 1 tsp dried oregano
- 3 cup fresh lemon juice
- Salt and ground black pepper to taste

Instructions

1. Wash and slice broccoli into florets.
2. In a bowl, toss broccoli, finely chopped mushrooms and minced garlic with little olive oil.
3. Season with a dried oregano, salt, and pepper to taste. Pour with lemon juice and stir well.
4. Place the mushrooms/broccoli mixture in a greased Crock Pot.

5. Cover and cook on LOW for 4 - 5 hours.
6. Serve warm.

Servings: 6
Cooking Times
Total Time: 35 minutes
Nutrition Facts
Serving size: 1/6 of a recipe (7 ounces)
Percent daily values based on the Reference Daily Intake (RDI) for a 2000 calorie diet.
Nutrition information calculated from recipe ingredients.
Amount Per Serving
Calories 75,64
Calories From Fat (21%) 16,09
% Daily Value
Total Fat 1,88g 3%
Saturated Fat 0,83g 4%
Cholesterol 3,67mg 1%
Sodium 110,53mg 5%
Potassium 638,26mg 18%
Total Carbohydrates 10,99g 4%
Fiber 0,41g 2%
Sugar 0,54g
Protein 7,54g 15%

Spicy Cheese Spinach Dip (Crock Pot)

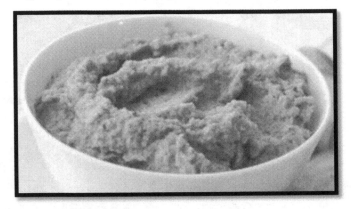

Ingredients

- 1 lb frozen spinach, chopped, thawed
- 1 cup hot cheese cream
- 1/2 cup bone broth (or water)
- 2 Tbsp dried minced onion
- 1/2 tsp of hot ground paprika

Instructions

1. Thaw, drain and squeeze the spinach; place in a colander (you can heat the spinach in a microwave oven for 1 - 2 minutes and then drain in a colander).
2. Combine all ingredients from the list in your Crock Pot; stir well.
3. Cover and cook on HIGH for about 2 hours.
4. Stir well and serve warm or cold.
5. Keep refrigerated.

Servings: 8

Cooking Times

Total Time: 2 hours and 10 minutes

Nutrition Facts

Serving size: 1/8 of a recipe (4 ounces)

Percent daily values based on the Reference Daily Intake (RDI) for a 2000 calorie diet.

Nutrition information calculated from recipe ingredients.

Amount Per Serving

Calories 129,59

Calories From Fat (75%) 97,48

% Daily Value

Total Fat 11,12g 17%

Saturated Fat 5,78g 29%

Cholesterol 31,9mg 11%

Sodium 356,15mg 15%

Potassium 225,27mg 6%

Total Carbohydrates 4,98g 2%

Fiber 2,19g 9%

Sugar 1,51g

Protein 4,23g 8%

Spicy Mushrooms with Parsley (Crock Pot)

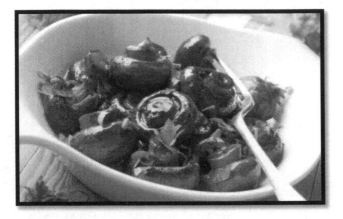

Ingredients

- 2 lbs fresh mushrooms, cleaned
- 1/2 cup Mayonnaise
- 1/4 cup water
- 1 Tbsp red pepper flakes
- 1/4 cup parsley finely chopped
- Kosher salt and black pepper to taste

Instructions

1. In your 4-quart Crock Pot, combine together the mushrooms, mayonnaise, water, red pepper flakes and finely chopped garlic. Stir well and cover lid.
2. Cook on LOW heat settings for 3 - 4 hours.
3. Serve warm.

Servings: 4

Cooking Times

Total Time: 6 hours

Nutrition Facts

Serving size: 1/4 of a recipe (9.6 ounces)

Percent daily values based on the Reference Daily Intake (RDI) for a 2000 calorie diet.

Nutrition information calculated from recipe ingredients.

Amount Per Serving

Calories 115,93

Calories From Fat (46%) 53,58

% Daily Value

Total Fat 6,18g 10%

Saturated Fat 1,04g 5%

Cholesterol 6,72mg 2%

Sodium 44,68mg 2%

Potassium 744,95mg 21%

Total Carbohydrates 8,11g 4%

Fiber 2,39g 10%

Sugar 5,7g

Protein 7,2g 14%

Spinach and Swiss chard with Almonds (Crock Pot)

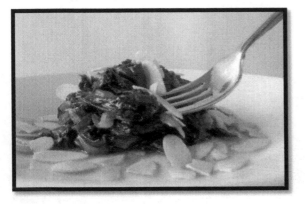

Ingredients

- 1 lb raw spinach leaves
- 1 lb Swiss chard raw
- 1/4 cup extra-virgin olive oil
- 3 cups water
- 1/2 cup toasted almond slivers
- Salt and black ground pepper to taste

Instructions

1. Wash well the spinach and the Swiss chard.
2. Remove the tough stems of Swiss chard and cut the tender stems and leaves torn into 2" pieces.
3. Pour the olive oil in your Crock Pot and place the spinach and Swiss chard on the bottom.
4. Season salt and pepper and stir well.

5. Place the half of almonds and pour the water; stir well.
6. Cover and cook on LOW for 4 - 6 hours or cook on HIGH for 1 - 3 hours.
7. Taste and adjust seasonings.
8. Serve with remaining almonds on the top.

Servings: 6
Cooking Times
Total Time: 6 hours
Nutrition Facts
Serving size: 1/6 of a recipe (10 ounces)
Percent daily values based on the Reference Daily Intake (RDI) for a 2000 calorie diet.
Nutrition information calculated from recipe ingredients.
Amount Per Serving
Calories 77,27
Calories From Fat (47%) 36,4
% Daily Value
Total Fat 4,36g 7%
Saturated Fat 0,37g 2%
Total Carbohydrates 5,29g 2%
Fiber 3,84g 15%
Sugar 1,46g
Protein 5,2g 10%

Sweet Potato Puree with Mustard (Crock Pot)

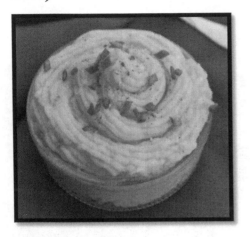

Ingredients

- 2 1/2 lbs of sweet potatoes peeled and cut into moderate pieces
- 2 Tbsp mustard
- ¼ cup butter grass-fed
- Salt and freshly ground pepper to taste

Instructions

1. Wash sweet potatoes well (do not dry off), and place directly on the bottom of the Crock Pot.
2. Cover and cook on HIGH for 3 - 4 hours or on LOW for 6-7 hours.
3. Let cool and peel the sweet potatoes.

4. Place the sweet potatoes in a large bowl and mash with a fork (do not use a blender because purée becomes sticky).
5. Add the mustard and the butter and stir well.
6. Season with salt and pepper to taste and give a good stir.
7. Serve immediately.

Servings: 6
Cooking Times
Total Time: 7 hours
Nutrition Facts
Serving size: 1/6 of a recipe (7 ounces)
Percent daily values based on the Reference Daily Intake (RDI) for a 2000 calorie diet.
Nutrition information calculated from recipe ingredients.
Amount Per Serving
Calories 37,43
Calories From Fat (95%) 35,52
% Daily Value
Total Fat 4,05g 6%
Saturated Fat 2,44g 12%
Total Carbohydrates 0,28g <1%
Fiber 0,17g <1%
Sugar 0,05g
Protein 0,27g <1%

SNACKS

Braised Zucchini and Basil with Parmesan (Crock Pot)

Ingredients

- 4 1/2 cups of zucchini sliced
- 1/2 cup of Olive oil
- 2 cloves of garlic
- 1 cup fresh basil leaves
- 1/4 cup Parmesan cheese
- Salt and pepper to taste

Instructions

1. Clean and peel the zucchini; cut into thick slices (or make a zucchini spaghetti with the help of mandolin).
2. Pour the olive oil on the bottom of your Crock Pot.
3. Add garlic, zucchini, chopped basil leaves and water (about one cup).
4. Season salt and pepper and stir well.
5. Cover and cook on LOW for 4-6 hours.
6. Transfer zucchini mixture to a serving plate.
7. Taste and adjust salt and pepper to taste.
8. Serve with grated or shaved Parmesan cheese.

Servings: 4

Cooking Times

Total Time: 6 hours

Nutrition Facts

Serving size: 1/4 of a recipe (7 ounces)

Percent daily values based on the Reference Daily Intake (RDI) for a 2000 calorie diet.

Nutrition information calculated from recipe ingredients.

Amount Per·Serving

Calories 294,01

Calories From Fat (88%) 258,83

% Daily Value

Total Fat 29,31g 45%

Saturated Fat 4,93g 25%

Cholesterol 5,5mg 2%

Sodium 107,94mg 4%

Potassium 409,46mg 12%

Total Carbohydrates 5,37g 2%

Fiber 1,6g 6%

Sugar 3,59g

Protein 4,52g 9%

Hot Bok Choi Salad with Sesame (Crock Pot)

Ingredients

- 2 bunch of Bok Choy, trimmed
- 1 small scallion finely chopped
- 1 cup water
- 2 Tbsp Olive oil
- 2 Tbsp Lemon juice
- Sesame seeds, lightly toasted

Instructions

1. Place the Bok Choi leaves in an empty sink. Cover with cold water and add a drop of vinegar. Swish everything around and let it stand for about 10 minutes. Then, lift the greens out of the water and strain.
2. Cut the leafy greens into bite-sized pieces.
3. Place the Bok Choy leaves in your Crock Pot and add the scallions, water, olive oil and lemon juice. Season salt and pepper and stir well.
4. Cover and cook on LOW for 4 hours.
5. Transfer the Bok Choy mixture to a serving plate.
6. Dress with salt and olive oil to taste.
7. Sprinkle some lemon juice and sesame and serve.

Servings: 4

Cooking Times

Total Time: 10 minutes

Nutrition Facts

Serving size: 1/4 of a recipe (8 ounces)

Percent daily values based on the Reference Daily Intake (RDI) for a 2000 calorie diet.

Nutrition information calculated from recipe ingredients.

Amount Per Serving

Calories 95,97

Calories From Fat (64%) 61,02

% Daily Value

Total Fat 6,91g 11%

Saturated Fat 0,98g 5%

Cholesterol 0mg 0%

Sodium 26,64mg 1%

Potassium 246,25mg 7%

Total Carbohydrates 5,56g 3%

Fiber 3,46g 14%

Sugar 2,56g

Protein 1,81g 4%

Hot Salad with Artichokes and Green Beans (Crock Pot)

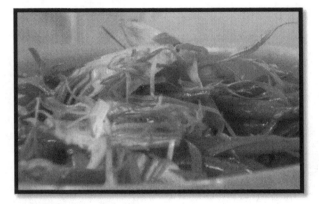

Ingredients

- 4 artichokes
- 1/2 lb green beans
- 3 lemons fresh juice
- 2 Tbsp Herbs mix (parsley, dill, thyme, sage...etc.)
- 1/2 cup olive oil
- Salt and black pepper to taste

Instructions

1. Clean the artichokes and immediately put them in a bowl of water and the lemon juice to avoid tanning. Then, gently cut into quarters.
2. Place the artichokes in your greased Crock Pot.
3. Add the green beans, salt and pepper and the herb mix.
4. Pour the water (about 2 cups) and stir.

5. Cover and cook on HIGH for 4 hours or on LOW for 6-7 hours, until artichokes are tender.
6. Taste and adjust salt, pepper, and herbs.
7. Serve hot with lemon juice.

Servings: 6
Cooking Times
Total Time: 7 hours
Nutrition Facts
Serving size: 1/6 of a recipe (6.5 ounces)
Percent daily values based on the Reference Daily Intake (RDI) for a 2000 calorie diet.
Nutrition information calculated from recipe ingredients.
Amount Per Serving
Calories 217,9
Calories From Fat (74%) 161,57
% Daily Value
Total Fat 18,29g 28%
Saturated Fat 2,55g 13%
Cholesterol 0mg 0%
Total Carbohydrates 9,72g 5%
Fiber 5,76g 23%
Sugar 2,83g
Protein 3,62g 7%

Savory Cauliflower Cream (Crock Pot)

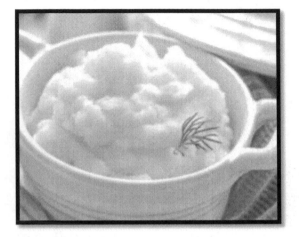

Ingredients

- 1 lb of cauliflower
- 2 cloves garlic pressed
- 2 cups water
- 3 Tbsp Olive oil
- 3 Tbsp butter (preferably grass-fed)
- Salt and pepper

Instructions

1. Lay the cauliflower florets in your Crock Pot and pour the oil and water. Season the salt and pepper.
2. Cover the lid and cook on LOW for 4 hours or until completely tender.
3. Transfer the cauliflower to your blender, and add the butter. Blend it until creamy.

4. Taste and adjust salt and pepper to taste.
5. Serve hot.

Servings: 4
Cooking Times
Total Time: 40 minutes
Nutrition Facts
Serving size: 1/4 of a recipe (9 ounces)
Percent daily values based on the Reference Daily Intake (RDI) for a 2000 calorie diet.
Nutrition information calculated from recipe ingredients.
Amount Per Serving
Calories 169,21
Calories From Fat (76%) 129,42
% Daily Value
Total Fat 14,89g 23%
Saturated Fat 1,8g 9%
Cholesterol 0mg 0%
Sodium 38,59mg 2%
Potassium 406,21mg 12%
Total Carbohydrates 7,64g 3%
Fiber 3,12g 12%
Sugar 2,54g`
Protein 3,95g 8%

Squash "Fingers" with Cinnamon-Cumin (Crock Pot)

Ingredients

- 1 lb butternut squash sliced
- 2 Tbsp extra virgin olive oil
- 1 1/2 tsp ginger, fresh, minced
- 1 tsp cinnamon
- 1/8 tsp ground cumin
- Salt to taste

Instructions

1. Line your Crock Pot with parchment paper.
2. Clean and peel the butternut squash, and slice with a mandolin slicer or with a knife.
3. Place sliced butternut squash in a bowl and set aside.
4. In a separate bowl, whisk olive oil, ginger, cinnamon and cumin seeds.
5. Pour the oil mixture over the butternut squash and toss well.
6. Place seasoned butternut squash in your Crock Pot.
7. Cover and cook on LOW for 4 - 6 hours.
8. Sprinkle with salt and cumin and serve.

Servings: 4

Cooking Times

Total Time: 1 hour and 40 minutes

Nutrition Facts

Serving size: 1/4 of a recipe (5 ounces)

Percent daily values based on the Reference Daily Intake (RDI) for a 2000 calorie diet.

Nutrition information calculated from recipe ingredients.

Amount Per Serving

Calories 52,64

Calories From Fat (2%) 1,14

% Daily Value

Total Fat 0,14g <1%

Saturated Fat 0,03g <1%

Cholesterol 0mg 0%

Sodium 4,83mg <1%

Potassium 404,4mg 12%

Total Carbohydrates 9,69g 5%

Fiber 2,48g 10%

Sugar 2,52g

Protein 1,16g 2%

Sweet Potato and Eggplant with Parmesan (Crock Pot)

Ingredients

- 1 lb sweet potatoes or yams
- 2 lbs eggplant
- 3/4 cup olive oil
- 1 bunch parsley, finely chopped
- 1 cup Parmesan cheese - grated
- Salt and ground pepper to taste

Instructions

1. Wash and clean the sweet potatoes.
2. Cut eggplants into thick slices, sprinkle them with salt and let them sit in a colander for half an hour.
3. Rinse the eggplant thoroughly and dry them.
4. Pour the olive oil in your Crock Pot and layer the eggplant slices.
5. Add the onions, 1 1/2 cups of water and salt pepper; stir well.
6. Cover and cook on HIGH for 4 - 5 hours or on LOW for 6 - 8 hours.
7. Taste and adjust seasonings per taste.
8. Serve hot with Parmesan on top.

Servings: 6

Cooking Times

Total Time: 8 hours and 10 minutes

Nutrition Facts

Serving size: 1/6 of a recipe (10 ounces)

Percent daily values based on the Reference Daily Intake (RDI) for a 2000 calorie diet.

Nutrition information calculated from recipe ingredients.

Amount Per Serving

Calories 398,87

Calories From Fat (82%) 328,55

% Daily Value

Total Fat 37,25g 57%

Saturated Fat 10,66g 53%

Cholesterol 26,33mg 9%

Sodium 176,58mg 7%

Potassium 423,24mg 12%

Total Carbohydrates 7,05g 3%

Fiber 5,35g 21%

Sugar 3,58g

Protein 8,87g 18%

Traditional Greek Tourlos (Crock Pot)

Ingredients

- 2 eggplants
- 1/2 lb zucchini sliced
- 4 cloves garlic, halved lengthwise
- 1 Tbsp fresh mint, oregano and basil leaves finely chopped.
- 1/4 cup of olive oil
- salt and freshly ground black pepper

Instructions

1. Cut the eggplants into slices, put them in a strainer, and sprinkle with salt; let rest for 30 minutes.
2. Rinse and drain them well and place in oiled Crock Pot.
3. Cut the zucchini into slices and place with halved garlic in your Crock Pot.
4. Season generously with herbs and salt the pepper.
5. Pour the oil and one cup water and stir well.
6. Cover the lid and cook on LOW for about 2-3 hours.
7. Taste, adjust salt and pepper and serve hot.

Servings: 5

Cooking Times

Total Time: 3 hours and 20 minutes

Nutrition Facts

Serving size: 1/5 of a recipe (8.5 ounces)

Percent daily values based on the Reference Daily Intake (RDI) for a 2000 calorie diet.

Nutrition information calculated from recipe ingredients.

Amount Per Serving

Calories 150,95

Calories From Fat (66%) 99,7

% Daily Value

Total Fat 11,31g 17%

Saturated Fat 1,59g 8%

Cholesterol 0mg 0%

Sodium 8,02mg <1%

Potassium 551,3mg 16%

Total Carbohydrates 7,69g 4%

Fiber 6,76g 27%

Sugar 4,46g

Protein 2,56g 5%

Warm Collard greens and Kalamata Olives Salad (Crock Pot)

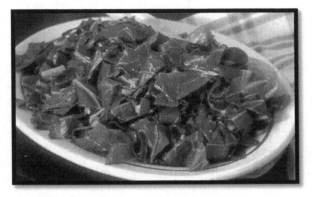

Ingredients

- 3 - 4 bunch of Collard greens, trimmed
- 1/2 cup Kalamata olives (green or black, or mix), sliced
- 2 Tbsp Olive oil
- Lemon juice, freshly squeezed
- Salt to taste
- 1 cup water

Instructions

1. Clean well the Collard greens; wash them in a sink, changing water three or four times, or until you don't see any grit in the water.
2. Place the Collard greens in the oiled Crock Pot along with all other ingredients from the list (except Olives).
3. Pour water and cover.

4. Cook on LOW for 6 hours.
5. Remove the Collard greens on a serving plate.
6. Add chopped olives and stir lightly.
7. Dress salad with salt, lemon juice, and olive oil before serving.

Servings: 2
Cooking Times
Total Time: 20 minutes
Nutrition Facts
Serving size: 1/2 of a recipe (10.5 ounces)
Percent daily values based on the Reference Daily Intake (RDI) for a 2000 calorie diet.
Nutrition information calculated from recipe ingredients.
Amount Per Serving
Calories 191,3
Calories From Fat (79%) 150,39
% Daily Value
Total Fat 17,14g 26%
Saturated Fat 2,37g 12%
Total Carbohydrates 7,8g 3%
Fiber 4,41g 18%
Sugar 3,27g
Protein 1,94g 4%

White Savory Vegetable Cream (Crock Pot)

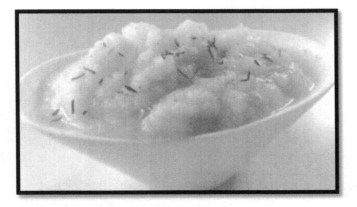

Ingredients

- 2 heads of Bok Choy, stems
- 1 leek finely chopped
- 1 lb cauliflower florets
- 2 Tbsp olive oil
- Salt and black ground pepper to taste

Instructions

1. Wash and chop all vegetables, and lay on the greased bottom of your Crock Pot.
2. Cover and cook on LOW setting for 1 1/2 - 2 hours.
3. Transfer vegetable (in bunches) in a blender, and blend until smooth and creamy.
4. Taste and adjust salt and pepper to taste. Serve warm.

Servings: 4

Cooking Times

Total Time: 25 minutes

Nutrition Facts

Serving size: 1/4 of a recipe (11.5 ounces)

Percent daily values based on the Reference Daily Intake (RDI) for a 2000 calorie diet.

Nutrition information calculated from recipe ingredients.

Amount Per Serving

Calories 101,59

Calories From Fat (62%) 62,91

% Daily Value

Total Fat 7,13g 11%

Saturated Fat 1,01g 5%

Cholesterol 0mg 0%

Sodium 38,61mg 2%

Potassium 379,18mg 11%

Total Carbohydrates 6,78g 3%

Fiber 2,67g 11%

Sugar 3,03g

Protein 2,51g 5%

Yams Puree with Almond-Cinnamon (Crock Pot)

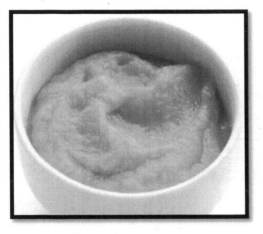

Ingredients

- 6 yams peeled and cut into small cubes
- 1 cup coconut milk (canned)
- 2-3 Tbsp Stevia (optional)
- 1/4 cup almond butter
- 1 1/2 tsp cinnamon

Instructions

1. Peel the skin off the yams and cut into small pieces.
2. Rinse the yam pieces in cold water.
3. Stir the almond butter, one tablespoon of coconut milk, Stevia and cinnamon in a mixing bowl.
4. Lay yams in the bottom of your Slow Cooker.
5. Pour the almond butter mixture over yams.

6. Cover and cook on LOW about 6-8 hours.
7. When ready, use a potato masher and beat until creamy and smooth.
8. Pour coconut milk and give a good stir with the spoon.
9. Serve.

Servings: 6

Cooking Times

Total Time: 8 hours

Nutrition Facts

Serving size: 1/6 of a recipe (6 ounces)

Percent daily values based on the Reference Daily Intake (RDI) for a 2000 calorie diet.

Nutrition information calculated from recipe ingredients.

Amount Per Serving

Calories 123,95

Calories From Fat (66%) 82,1

% Daily Value

Total Fat 9,81g 15%

Saturated Fat 4g 20%

Total Carbohydrates 6,78g 3%

Fiber 1,43g 6%

Sugar 4,22g

Protein 2,61g 5%

SWEETS

Chocolate Ducat Cake (Crock Pot)

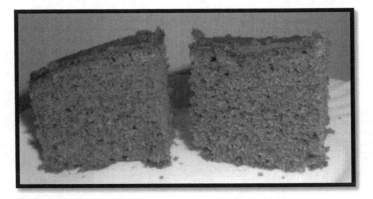

Ingredients

- 8 egg yolks
- 3/4 cup Stevia (or to taste)
- 1/3 cup cocoa powder unsweetened
- 2 1/4 cups heavy cream
- 1 1/2 tsp vanilla

Instructions

1. Whisk eggs yolks, Stevia and a pinch of salt.
2. Add the cream and vanilla and whisk until smooth.
3. Add the cocoa powder and continue to whisk.
4. Pour the batter into your oiled Crock Pot.
5. Cover and cook on LOW for 3 hours. The cake is ready when there are no wet spots on top and has pulled away from the sides of the crock

6. Let cool completely on room temperature.
7. Slice and serve.

Servings: 6
Cooking Times
Total Time: 15 minutes
Nutrition Facts
Serving size: 1/6 of a recipe (3.7 ounces)
Percent daily values based on the Reference Daily Intake (RDI) for a 2000 calorie diet.
Nutrition information calculated from recipe ingredients.
Amount Per Serving
Calories 221,96
Calories From Fat (84%) 186,88
% Daily Value
Total Fat 21,64g 33%
Saturated Fat 12,29g 61%
Cholesterol 241,5mg 81%
Sodium 26,09mg 1%
Potassium 126mg 4%
Total Carbohydrates 4,99g 2%
Fiber 1,58g 6%
Sugar 0,36g
Protein 4,49g 9%

Coconut Dream Cake (Crock Pot)

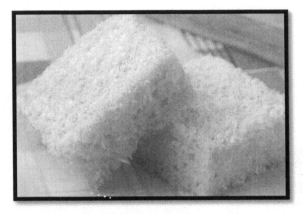

Ingredients

- 1 cup of coconut oil melted
- 2 1/4 cup of coconut flour
- 1/2 cup coconut milk canned
- 1 cup Stevia (or to taste)
- 3 eggs

Instructions

1. Beat melted coconut oil and Stevia with the mixer.
2. Add eggs one by one and stir well after each egg.
3. Combine the coconut flour, one teaspoon of baking powder and a pinch of salt in a bowl.
4. Gradually, add the coconut milk, combine with the coconut oil mixture until the flour is just mixed.
5. Grease the bottom of your Crock Pot with coconut oil, and line with baking paper.

6. Spread dough evenly on baking paper.
7. Close and cook on HIGH about 1 - 1 1/2 hours.
8. When ready, remove from the cooker and let cool for 20 minutes on the room temperature.
9. Serve.

Servings: 8
Cooking Times
Total Time: 1 hour and 50 minutes
Nutrition Facts
Serving size: 1/8 of a recipe (5 ounces)
Percent daily values based on the Reference Daily Intake (RDI) for a 2000 calorie diet.
Nutrition information calculated from recipe ingredients.
Amount Per Serving
Calories 324
Calories From Fat (86%) 278,13
% Daily Value
Total Fat 32,29g 50%
Saturated Fat 27,04g 135%
Total Carbohydrates 6,15g 3%
Fiber 0,74g 3%
Sugar 5,07g
Protein 3,2g 6%

Easy Almond-Lemon Cake (Crock Pot)

Ingredients

- 2 cups blanched whole almonds
- 6 large eggs, preferably organic
- 1 1/4 cups Stevia (or to taste)
- 4 drops almond extract
- Grated zest of 1 lemon
- Non-stick cooking spray

Instructions

1. Oil the bottom of your Crock Pot.
2. Grind the almonds in a food processor.
3. Whisk the egg yolks with the Stevia until smooth.
4. Pour the almond extract and lemon zest.
5. Add the ground almonds and stir well.
6. In a separate mixing bowl, beat the egg whites until stiff peaks form.
7. Combine the egg whites mixture with the egg yolks mixture and stir well.
8. Pour the cake mixture in a prepared Crock Pot and sprinkle with finely chopped almonds.
9. Cover and cook on HIGH for 1 1/2 - 2 hours.
10. Let cool and serve.

Servings: 8

Cooking Times

Total Time: 2 hours

Nutrition Facts

Serving size: 1/8 of a recipe (4.2 ounces)

Percent daily values based on the Reference Daily Intake (RDI) for a 2000 calorie diet.

Nutrition information calculated from recipe ingredients.

Amount Per Serving

Calories 259,45

Calories From Fat (69%) 178,34

% Daily Value

Total Fat 21,53g 33%

Saturated Fat 2,56g 13%

Cholesterol 139,5mg 47%

Sodium 54,33mg 2%

Potassium 298,59mg 9%

Total Carbohydrates 6,27g 3%

Fiber 3,84g 15%

Sugar 1,87g

Protein 11,99g 24%

Sweet Cinnamon-Vanilla Almonds (Crock Pot)

Ingredients

- 1 1/2 cups Stevia
- 3 Tbsp cinnamon
- 1 egg white
- 2 tsp vanilla
- 3 cups almonds

Instructions

1. Combine together Stevia and cinnamon in a large bowl.
2. In a separate bowl, whisk the egg white and vanilla until it is frothy.
3. Combine Stevia mixture with egg white mixture.
4. Add the almonds and coat thoroughly.
5. Oil a 4-quart Crock Pot.
6. Place the cinnamon almond mixture to the pot. Stir until the cinnamon mixture is combined well.
7. Cover and cook on LOW 3 - 4 hours stirring every 20 minutes.
8. Transfer the almonds to a baking sheet lined with parchment paper and spread the almonds onto the sheet to cool.
9. Serve and enjoy!!

Servings: 6

Cooking Times

Total Time: 4 hours and 10 minutes

Nutrition Facts

Serving size: 1/6 of a recipe (3.9 ounces)

Percent daily values based on the Reference Daily Intake (RDI) for a 2000 calorie diet.

Nutrition information calculated from recipe ingredients.

Amount Per Serving

Calories 248,72

Calories From Fat (65%) 160,9

% Daily Value

Total Fat 20,01g 31%

Saturated Fat 1,52g 8%

Cholesterol 0mg 0%

Sodium 10,16mg <1%

Potassium 312,6mg 9%

Total Carbohydrates 9,61g 5%

Fiber 7g 28%

Sugar 1,87g

Protein 9,33g 19%

Made in the USA
Lexington, KY
27 December 2017